Improving
FLEXIBILITY

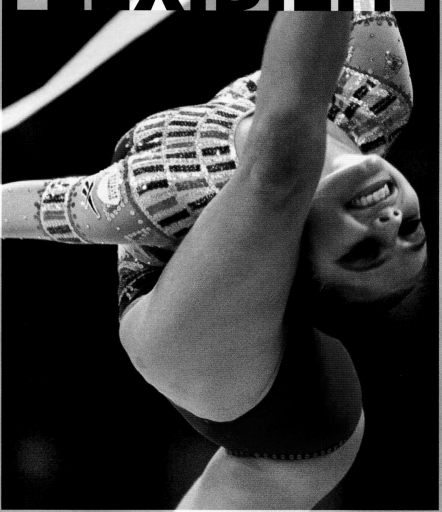

Paul Mason

PowerKiDS press™

New York

Published in 2011 by The Rosen Publishing Group Inc.
29 East 21st Street, New York, NY 10010

First Edition

Editor: Julia Adams
Designer: Tim Mayer, Mayer Media
Proofreader and Indexer: Claire Shanahan
Picture Researcher: Kathy Lockley
Consultant: Professor John Brewer

Library of Congress Cataloging-in-Publication Data

Mason, Paul.
 Improving flexibility / by Paul Mason. -- 1st ed.
   p. cm. -- (Training for sports)
 ISBN 978-1-4488-3299-6 (library binding)
 1. Stretching exercises. 2. Physical education and training.
 3. Joints--Range of motion. I. Title.
 GV711.5.M37 2011
 613.7'1--dc22
                           2010024359

Manufactured in China
CPSIA Compliance Information: Batch #WAW1102PK: For Further Information
contact Rosen Publishing, New York, New York at 1-800-237-9932

Picture acknowledgements
EITAN ABRAMOVICH/AFP/Getty Images: 22
Ben Blankenburg/iStock Photography: 6
FRANCK CAMHI/Alamy: 25
Jakub Cejpek/Shutterstock: COVER
Directphoto.org/Alamy: 26
Epic Stock/Shutterstock: background throughout
Greg Epperson/Shutterstock: background throughout
FAN travelstock/Alamy: 12
ingret/Shutterstock: background throughout
Julian Finney/Getty Images: 9
Stu Forster/Getty Images: 19T
John Fryer/Alamy: 24
AdrianHillman/iStock images: folios throughout
hkannn /Shutterstock: 8
Robbie Jack/Corbis: 5
Herbert Kratky /Shutterstock: COVER (small, middle)
Nick Laham/Getty Images: 11
Sandra Mu/Getty Images: 18
PA Photos/Topfoto/Topfoto.co.uk: 27
Gabe Palmer/Alamy: 14
Mana Photo /Shutterstock: COVER (small, top)
Edyta Pawlowska /Shutterstock: COVER (small, bottom)
Mike Powell/Allsport/Getty Images: title page, 23
Clive Rose/Getty Images: 19B
Joanna T./Alamy: 10
John Terence Turner/Alamy: 4
Asya Verzhbinsky/ArenaPAL/TopFoto.co.uk: 15
© 2010 Beth Wald/Beth Wald Photography: 13
Troy Wayrynen/New Sport/Corbis: 7

Photography: Andy Crawford (16–17; 20–21; 28–29)

Disclaimer
In the preparation of this book, care has been exercised with
regard to advice, activities and techniques. However, when
the reader is learning or engaged in a sport or utilizing a piece
of equipment, the reader should get advice from an expert
and follow the manufacturer's instructions. The publisher
cannot be, and is not liable for, any loss or injury the reader
may sustain.

Contents

Bending Your Body

Your probably have friends who are more bendy, or flexible, than everyone else. Maybe they find it easier to touch their toes. Maybe they have especially snaky hips on the dance floor! Of course, flexibility isn't only useful at a party—it's also important in almost all sports.

What Is Flexibility?

Flexibility is the ability to move your joints through a wide range of movement. The main joints are the ankles, knees, hips, waist, shoulders, elbows, and neck, but there are many more. In fact, the human body contains over a hundred joints. Joints can be bent and straightened by your muscles, which pull on them to make them move.

Why Is Flexibility Important?

Flexibility is important in sports because an athlete's flexibility affects their skills and technique. Just think of these two examples:

- Imagine you're playing soccer, and a pass comes your way. It's not a very good pass, so you need to stretch out your leg to stop the ball. With good flexibility, this will not be a problem. But if your flexibility is poor, the ball might get past you—or it might even just touch your toes, before dribbling across the line for a goal!

- Suppose you want to learn how to do the splits at a gymnastics class. As long as both your hip joints are flexible, this should be possible. Otherwise, you will not manage it.

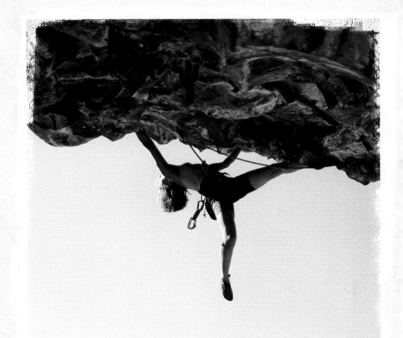

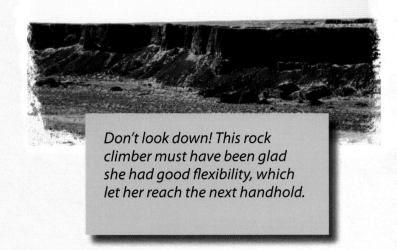

Don't look down! This rock climber must have been glad she had good flexibility, which let her reach the next handhold.

4

In almost every sport, to have first-rate skills and technique, you must be able to move your joints in exactly the right way. This means you need to be flexible. Otherwise, you will not be as good as the people who are very flexible!

Some people are born bendy; others have to work at it. The good news is that, with the right help, everyone can improve their flexibility.

Sylvie Guillem's long legs and powerful technique helped her to revolutionize ballet.

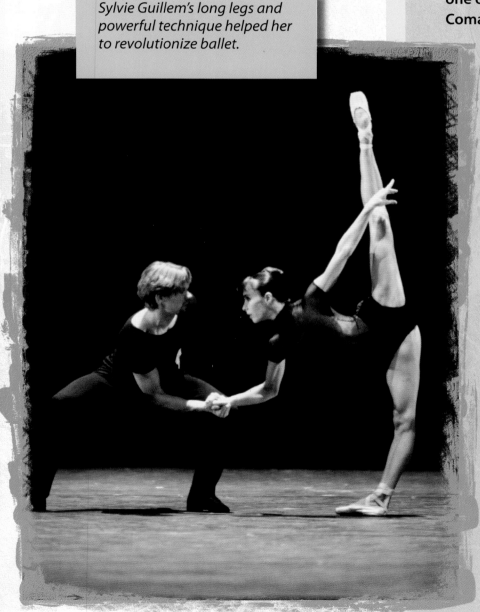

Sylvie Guillem

Sport: Ballet, dance

Country: France

Born: February 23, 1965

Guillem's first sport was gymnastics: one of her heroes is the gymnast Nadia Comaneci. But at the age of 11, as part of her gymnastics training, Guillem went to a dance class. She was quickly hooked.

Soon, Guillem was training at the Paris Opera Ballet School. Four years later, she was invited to join the Paris Opera Ballet Company. Then, in 1984, Guillem was talent-spotted by the famous dancer Rudolf Nureyev. She became the Company's youngest-ever etoile, the highest rank of female dancer—she was just 19 years old.

What made Guillem stand out was that she is very tall and very strong. Tall girls were not usually welcome in ballet, but Guillem's talent was so great it could not be ignored. She went on to dance with great success all around the world, and is still a freelance dancer with some of the world's top companies.

Flexibility in Sports

All sportspeople need to have good flexibility, but it is more crucial to success in some sports than others. Darts players, for example, would probably agree that flexibility isn't at the top of their list of training requirements. But flexibility is a must for gymnasts, for instance, who require fast, accurate positioning of their whole body.

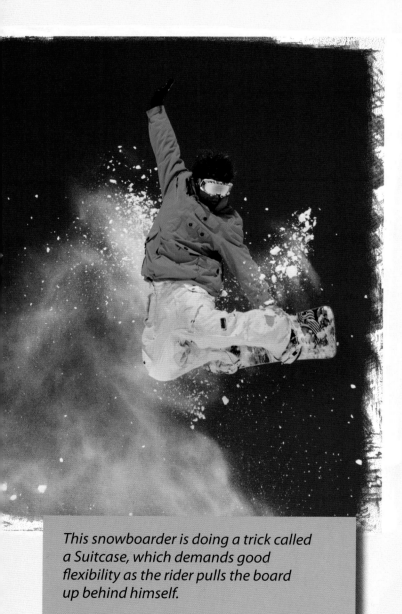

This snowboarder is doing a trick called a Suitcase, which demands good flexibility as the rider pulls the board up behind himself.

Sports that Demand Flexibility

Sports activities where flexibility makes the difference between success and failure include:

- dance
- gymnastics (including trampolining)
- diving
- martial arts such as judo, tae kwon do, karate, and boxing
- rock climbing.

There are many other sports where improving your flexibility leads to better performance: all sports that involve running, swimming, or cycling, and every racket sport, for example.

Technical Ability

A high level of flexibility is very important in sports that rely on specialist, technical movements. Good examples are the high jump and pole vault. In each of these, the athlete approaches the jump from the front. Then, as part of their technique to help convert their forward movement into upward movement, they twist around. The twist they make is not one people normally do. This means the athletes have to work on their flexibility to improve their twisting ability.

PROFESSIONAL PROFILE

Chris Sharma

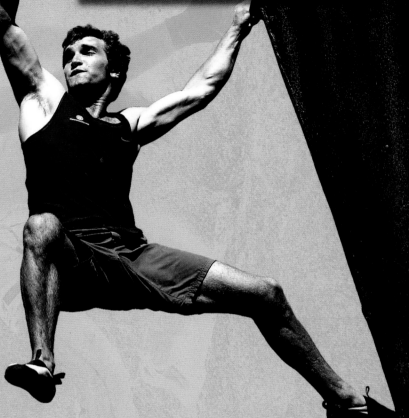

Sport: Rock climbing

Country: France

Born: April 23, 1981

Chris Sharma has been called the world's best rock climber. He has climbed three of the world's hardest known routes. Some of his climbs are so difficult that no one else has been able to repeat them.

Sharma started climbing at the age of 12. Two years later, when he was 14, he won the U.S. National Championship for bouldering. Bouldering is a form of climbing at low level, which features extraordinarily difficult maneuvers. Reaching the holds and then pulling up on them requires great strength and flexibility.

Sharma's most famous climbs include:
- The first successful climb of The Mandala, one of the world's hardest bouldering challenges.
- Realization/Biographie: the world's first climb to be graded 5.15a.
- Witness The Fitness: an even harder boulder challenge than Mandala.
- Jumbo Love and Golpe de Estadio: both possibly graded 5.15b, though by 2009, no one had repeated them to confirm the difficulty.

Injury Prevention

Having good flexibility makes it less likely that a sportsperson will get injured, in both training and competition. Flexibility is controlled by the body's muscles, the shape of the joints, and the tissues that connect the two. Lack of flexibility places these under strain, especially if they are asked to perform movements outside their normal range. This increases the chances of injury. Improving your flexibility makes it less likely that this kind of injury will happen.

Joint Structure

Improving flexibility means making your joints work better, over as wide a range of movement as possible. When aiming to do this, you need to know how joints work. That way, you understand what is happening when you do flexibility exercises. You also see how dangerous it can be to overstress a joint.

Types of Joint

A joint is a place where two bones meet. There are three major kinds of joint:

Fibrous joints

Fibrous joints barely move at all. Your skull, for example, is made up of several plates of bone. If they were able to move much, it would be very upsetting (and dangerous)! Instead, the plates are linked together by tough tissue.

Cartilaginous Joints

Cartilaginous joints have limited movement. The best example is the joints in your spine. Each spine bone is connected to the next with a pad of material called cartilage.

Synovial joints

Synovial joints allow a relatively wide range of movement, and it is these that are most connected to our flexibility. Examples include the foot, knee, hip, wrist, and elbow joints.

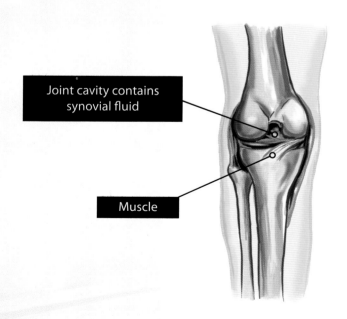

Joint cavity contains synovial fluid

Muscle

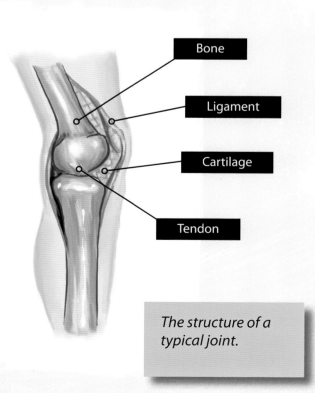

Bone

Ligament

Cartilage

Tendon

The structure of a typical joint.

Synovial Joint Structure

Typical synovial joints are made up of five main elements:

1) The bones, specifically the bone ends.

2) Cartilage, a pad of tough material that helps protect the bone ends.

3) Synovial fluid, inside a membrane. This sits inside the joint between the two bones, providing lubrication (a little like oil on a bike chain) and helping to keep the cartilage in good condition.

4) Ligaments, tough fibers that support the joint and help it keep its shape. Ligaments can be stretched to make them more flexible, but not too much. Loose ligaments will not keep the joint in shape properly, which makes injury more likely.

5) Tendon, which attaches the bone to the muscles that move it.

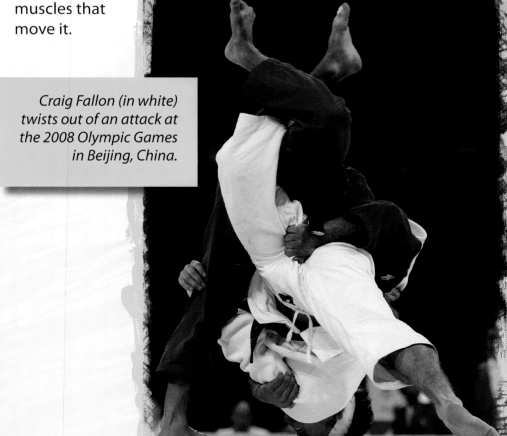

Craig Fallon (in white) twists out of an attack at the 2008 Olympic Games in Beijing, China.

Craig FALLON

Sport: Judo

Country: UK

Born: December 18, 1982

Craig Fallon is one of the world's top judoka, or judo fighters. He competes in the 130-lb. (60-kg) division. Fallon is famous for his slippery ability to escape from throws and other attacks by his opponents.

Fallon's career highlights include:

- Gold medal at the Commonwealth Games in 2002, and silver medals at both European and World Championships in 2003.
- In 2005, he was crowned world champion in Cairo, Egypt. Fallon was only the third British man ever to be world champion.
- In 2006, at the European Championships in Finland, Fallon again took gold. He was only the second British fighter ever to hold world and European titles at the same time.
- Fallon also won the 2007 Men's World Cup, a season-long points competition based on results at top-level competitions.

Muscles and Flexibility

Your muscles control how your joints move. They do this by bunching up, which pulls the muscle ends together. The ends are attached to tendons, which are attached to the joint. When a muscle contracts, the joint moves. When a different muscle bunches up and the first one relaxes, the joint moves in another direction.

Moving Joints and Increasing Flexibility

Muscles act in two main ways when controlling your joints. Muscles that contract are the ones causing movement. Muscles that relax are the ones that oppose movement: they stop the joint moving too far, but also limit its flexibility.

Your muscles have other controls and safety devices to protect joints. The body's central nervous system makes sure that when one muscle pulls, the other relaxes. There are also hard-wired reactions stopping relaxing muscles overstretching, and protecting contracting muscles from too-heavy loads or too-fast movement.

All these controls can be affected by training. The muscles become better able to relax when in opposing-movement mode. This increases flexibility and the joint's range of movement.

Limits on Flexibility

Flexibility is limited both by our own bodies and by outside factors. It is important to bear these in mind when stretching. They may mean you cannot stretch as far as the person next to you:

- Physical differences, such as the shape of bones, can limit movement. Everyone's joints have the same basic structure, but there are big differences between individuals' joints. The differences may be caused by physical exercise: for instance, girls who do ballet from an early age usually have flexible hips. Joint differences may be things you are born with, or they may be caused by injuries.

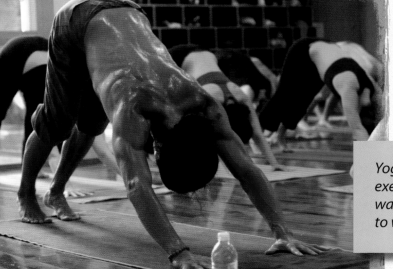

Yoga classes (and other stretching exercises) are more effective in a warm place. The heat helps the joints to work more easily.

- Joints and muscles will be stiffer if recovering after exercise.
- Younger people are generally more flexible than older ones; and females are usually more flexible than males.
- Flexibility is also affected by the temperature: warmer temperature = increased flexibility.
- Most people are more flexible in the afternoon and evening than the morning.

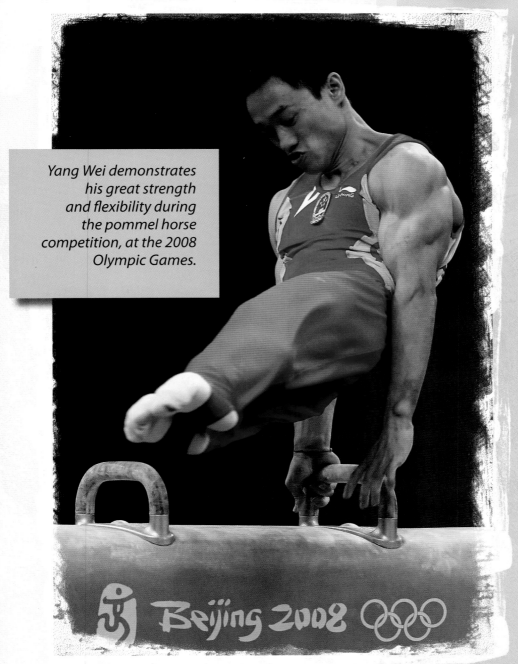

Yang Wei demonstrates his great strength and flexibility during the pommel horse competition, at the 2008 Olympic Games.

PROFESSIONAL PROFILE

Yang Wei

Sport: Artistic gymnastics

Country: China

Born: February 8, 1980

Yang Wei is one of the world's top gymnasts, famous for his ability to combine strength and flexibility. This allows him to include techniques with a very high difficulty rating in his routines.

Yang (his last name is Yang, his first name is Wei) came to the world's attention when he won an all-around silver, and team gold, at the 2000 Sydney Olympics. His other career highlights include:

- All-around silver and team gold at the World Championships in 2003.
- Gold in the team, all-around, and parallel bars at the 2006 World Championships, and team and all-around titles at the 2007 World Championships.
- All-around and team gold at the 2008 Olympic Games, plus silver in the rings and fifth in the pommel horse.

Flexibility and Technique

Imagine you're a gymnast on a balance beam. You want to do a backward somersault, which means falling backward with an arched back, placing your hands on the 4-in.- (10-cm-) wide beam, and gracefully lifting your legs over to land on the far end of the beam. (Don't try this at home!) Unless you're very flexible, you won't have a chance of doing it.

The backward somersault on a beam is an extreme example of how without flexibility, it is impossible to have good technique. But most other sports also require particular muscles and joints to work as efficiently as possible.

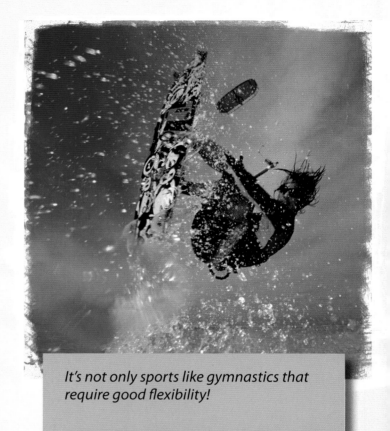

It's not only sports like gymnastics that require good flexibility!

Running Sports

Running places particular demands on the legs and feet:

1) When your heel strikes the ground, one set of muscles stops your foot slapping down on the ground. Another set stops your foot from flattening too much. If either of these sets of muscles is too tight, it causes shin pain.

2) Midway through a running stride, muscles in your leg and hip work to drive you forward. If any of these are tight, knee pain can often result.

3) Then as you push off the ground, calf muscles and hamstrings control the foot and hip. If either of these is tight, injuries become more likely.

4) Finally, muscles in your hips lift your leg through. If these lack flexibility, it may cause lower back pain.

It is easy to see from this why it is so important for runners to have good flexibility, and to warm up their muscles before working hard. (See page 22 for more on warming up.)

Other Sports

Like running, other sports activities place specific demands on the muscles and joints. Swimmers and throwers need flexible shoulders and torsos. Gymnasts need flexible backs (and everything else!). Dancers need flexible legs and backs.

Top athletes work on overall flexibility, but they and their coaches pay special attention to the muscles they use while performing key techniques.

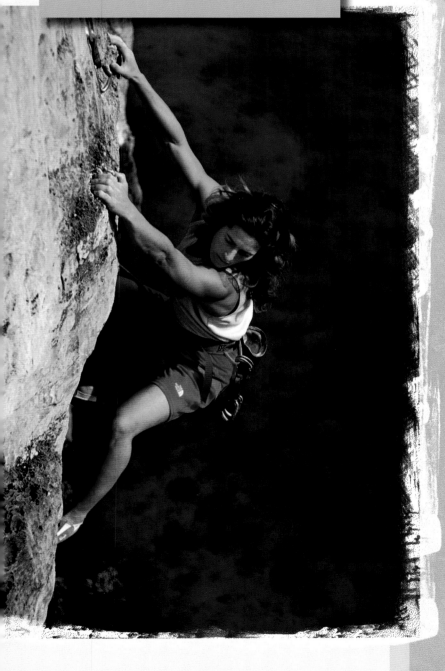

Lynn Hill climbs one of many new routes on the beautiful limestone pillars of Ha Long Bay, Vietnam.

Lynn Hill

Sport: Rock climbing

Country: U.S.A.

Born: 1961

Lynn Hill is one the best-known climbers in the world. Her famous climbs in Yosemite National Park have put her among the best climbers ever, male or female.

Hill only started climbing at the age of 14. She was soon setting new standards: at first for female climbers, then for climbers of either sex. Hill's amazing strength, fitness, and flexibility have kept her at the top of the climbing world for many years:

- In 1979, Hill became the first woman ever to establish a new climb at the grade 5.12+/5.13, Ophir Broke, in Colorado.
- She became the first woman to climb at grade 5.14, with an ascent of Masse Critique in France in 1991.
- In 1993, Hill and a partner became the first people ever to climb The Nose, one of Yosemite's most famous routes, using only natural holds. A year later, Hill went one better and climbed The Nose alone, in under 24 hours. It would be ten years before either feat was repeated.

How to Stretch

Stretching exercises help sportspeople to improve their flexibility. They do this by encouraging a greater range of movement in muscles and joints than they previously managed. Because of this, stretching carries a risk of injury. It pays to follow some basic rules when working on stretches.

Never Make it Painful!

The key rule for working on flexibility is that if any stretch becomes even slightly painful, you should stop immediately. This applies to both stretches you perform alone and to stretches done with the help of someone else.

Warm Up

The body responds best to stretches once it is warm, and the muscles have been used, but not strained. It is a good idea to warm up before beginning a set of stretching exercises. Do some light exercise for 5–10 minutes, ideally using the muscles and joints you are aiming to work on. Even athletes doing stretches as *part* of their warm-up should do some light exercise first.

By the time you start stretching, you should be sweating lightly. Wear loose clothes that will keep in body heat.

Ease into the Stretch

Always ease into a stretch slowly. Never "bounce" your body into a stretch to try and get farther into it. Stretch the muscle while breathing out. If you have to breathe in, stop stretching until you are ready to breath out again. This is a useful way of extending a stretch slightly beyond your usual position, without it feeling uncomfortable.

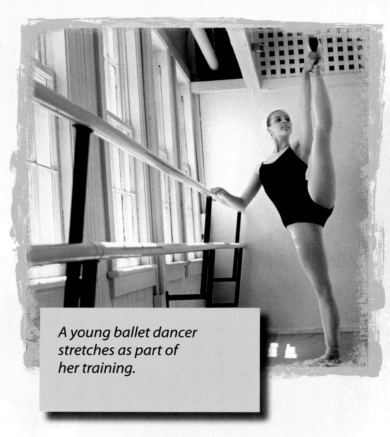

A young ballet dancer stretches as part of her training.

Holding Your Position

If a stretch is being done as part of a flexibility session, most coaches suggest holding it for anything from 10–30 seconds. (If the stretch were part of a warm-up or cool-down, it would normally be held for a shorter time.) While holding your position, breathe normally and stay relaxed. When the time is up, gently ease out of the stretch and return to your starting position.

Carlos
ACOSTA

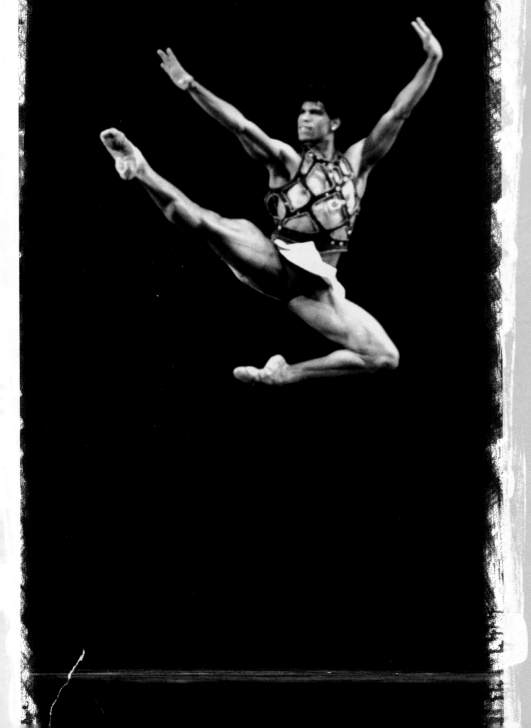

Carlos Acosta dancing in a UK Royal Ballet production. The Cuban is one of the biggest box-office attractions in dance.

Sport: Ballet dancer

Country: Cuba

Born: December 18, 1982

Carlos Acosta is one of the most famous and popular dancers in the world. His performances draw huge crowds, and there is even a ballet based on his own life.

Born in Havana, Cuba, Acosta once dreamed of being a professional soccer player. His father had different ideas, and sent him to ballet school. Within a few years, he had hit the headlines by winning the Prix de Lausanne, a dance competition aimed at discovering the world's greatest talents.

Today, Acosta's combination of power and flexibility is unusual even among dancers. He is known for his high, graceful leaps and strong technique. One newspaper reviewer described him as, "a dancer who slashes across space faster than anyone else, who [cuts] the air with shapes so clear and sharp they seem to throw off sparks."

Static Stretching

Static stretching involves easing yourself into a stretch. You stop as you begin to feel mild discomfort (NOT pain) in the antagonistic muscles (the ones that are supposed to be relaxing). Then you hold the position. Sometimes the position is held using another part of your body or a partner.

The Stretch Reflex

All muscles controlling our joints have a stretch reflex. This is a safety device to stop the muscle from stretching too far, and overextending the joint. Over time, stretching exercises will cause this stretch reflex to kick in later. This allows the muscles to extend slightly farther, and the joint to open slightly more, than before.

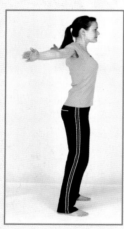

Chest Stretch

You should feel this stretch across your chest:

1) Stand tall, feet slightly more than shoulder-width apart, knees slightly bent.

2) Hold your arms straight out to the side, parallel to the ground, the palms of your hands facing forward.

3) Stretch your arms back as far as possible.

Upper Back Stretch

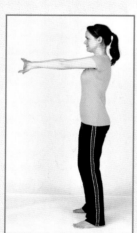

You should feel this stretch between your shoulder blades:

1) Do step 1) in the chest stretch.

2) Interlock your fingers, turn them inside-out, and push your hands away from your chest as far as possible. Allow your upper back to relax.

Shoulder Stretch

You should feel this stretch on the back and outside of your shoulder:

1) Do step 1) in the chest stretch.

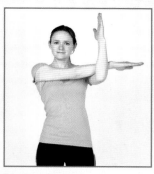

2) Place your straight right arm across your chest, parallel with the ground.

3) Lift your left arm up, and use your forearm to ease the right arm closer to your chest.

4) Repeat with your other arm.

Side Bends

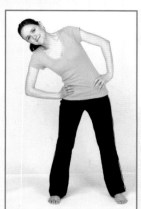

You should feel this stretch at the side of your body, below your rib cage.

1) Do step 1) of the chest stretch, but with your hands resting on your hips.

2) Bend slowly to one side, without leaning forward or backward—ONLY lean sideways.

3) Straighten up, then bend to the other side.

Hamstring Stretch

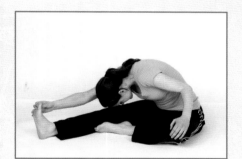

You should feel this stretch in your hamstrings:

1) Sit on the ground with your legs out in front of you in a comfortable V shape.

2) Bring the sole of your left foot in to rest against your right knee. Allow the left leg to lie relaxed on the ground.

3) Bend forward, keeping the back straight, to touch your right foot with your right hand. Rest your left hand on your left knee.

4) Relax, then repeat with the other leg.

Calf Stretch

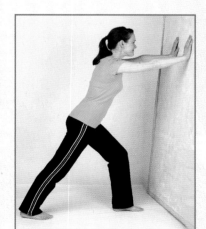

You should feel this stretch in the calf of your rear leg:

1) Stand facing a wall, with one leg slightly forward.

2) Put your hands flat against the wall at shoulder height.

3) Ease your back leg away from the wall, keeping it straight. Press your heel firmly into the floor.

4) Keep your hips parallel to the wall, and your back leg and spine in a straight line.

5) Relax, then repeat with the other leg.

Assisted Stretching

Assisted stretching is useful because, with the help of a partner, it encourages your body into positions it could not normally manage on its own. It also makes it possible to include an element of resistance training in the stretch.

Risk of Injury

Assisted stretching offers the greatest gains in flexibility in the shortest possible time. It does this because using a partner allows you to stretch the muscles farther than would otherwise be possible. But this also means that assisted stretching has the highest chance of injury through overstretching. These injuries are usually caused by the partner who is supposed to be helping.

When doing assisted stretching, it is crucial that your partner takes the risk of injury seriously, and never pushes the stretch too far. Top athletes only ever do this kind of stretch with an experienced, properly trained partner.

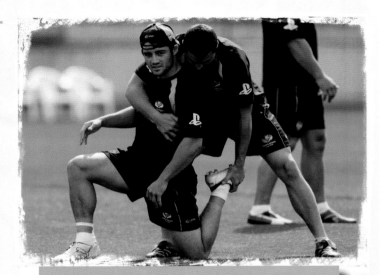

Cooper Cronk and an Australian rugby league teammate stretching before a game in new Zealand.

PNF Stretching

PNF stands for Proprioceptive Neuromuscular Facilitation. PNF stretching is a development of assisted stretching. Your partner not only helps you to achieve a stretch position, but also helps you to take the position farther. PNF stretching works by tensing the antagonistic muscle, then relaxing it further with the help of your partner:

1) First, you move into the stretch position, so that you feel the stretch sensation.

2) Your partner holds the limb steady in this position.

3) You push against your partner, tightening the antagonistic muscles. Your partner aims to stop the limb moving at all. Push for 6 to 10 seconds, then relax.

4) As you relax, your partner gently moves the limb farther into the stretch, stopping as you feel the stretch sensation again.

5) This is repeated 3 or 4 times, each time moving a little farther into the stretch position, before the stretch is released.

Mitchell Johnson of Australia bowls against England in a 2009 cricket international. It's clear from the position of his shoulders that cricket players need good flexibility.

Tom Daley

Sport: Diving
Country: UK
Born: May 21, 1994

Tom Daley shot to fame in 2007, when he and his diving partner, Callum Johnstone, won the silver medal at the Youth Olympics Festival. Daley had been given special permission to compete: the minimum age was 15, and he was only 12 years old.

In 2008, at the age of 13, Daley became the youngest person ever to win gold at the European Swimming Championships. At the 2008 Olympics, he and his new diving partner, Blake Aldridge, finished 8th.

A year later, at the 2009 World Championships in Rome, Daley surprised his competitors by taking the gold medal in the 10-meter diving competition. He was still only 15 years old, and this seemed unlikely to be his last medal at a major championship.

Tom Daley shows off a perfect pike position, while diving at a competition in Rome, Italy, in 2009.

Dynamic Stretching

How many times does a football player swing his or her leg back and then kick the ball during a game, or even a practice session? A hundred? Two hundred? So it's important that the player's muscles are able to stretch through the kick, and are warmed up ready to make passes the moment the game begins. One way to do this is by swinging their legs in a controlled way, to mimic the muscle movements made while kicking the ball. This kind of stretch is called dynamic stretching.

Dynamic stretching is useful for any sport that involves dynamic movement, from football to boxing, swimming, baseball, or dancing. Dynamic stretches such as the ones shown here are especially useful as part of a warm-up. (Static stretches are often used as part of a cool-down.) They should be done in a slow, controlled way, feeling relaxed and breathing steadily.

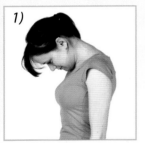
1)

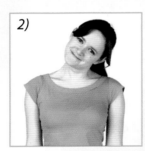
2)

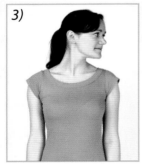
3)

Neck Mobility

Each of these neck exercises should be done 6–10 times:
1) Tuck your chin into your chest, and then lift your head back as far as possible.

2) Lower your left ear toward your left shoulder (DON'T lift your shoulder toward your ear!), then your right ear to your right shoulder.

3) Turn your chin to the side toward your left shoulder, then back to your right shoulder.

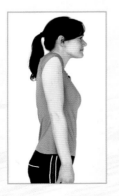
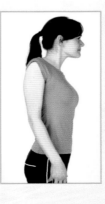

Shoulder Circles

1) Stand with your feet slightly more than shoulder-width apart and your knees slightly bent.

2) Lift your right shoulder toward your right ear, backward, down and up to your ear again, in a smooth action.

3) Repeat with the other shoulder.

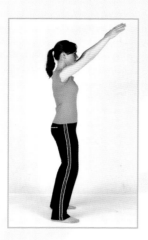
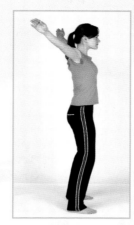

Arm Swings

Keep your arms and back straight when doing these swings. Repeat each 6–10 times:

1) Start as for step 1) of the shoulder circles.

2) Swing both arms continuously from an overhead position backward, down, and up.

3) Swing both arms out to your sides, then in to cross in front of your chest.

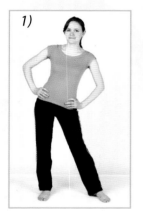
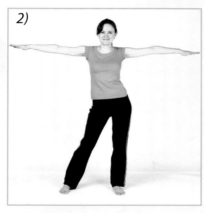

Hip Circles and Twists

Repeat each of these 10–12 times:

1) With your hands on your hips, stand with your feet a little wider apart than your shoulders. Make circles with your hips in a clockwise direction, then repeat counterclockwise.

2) With your arms out to the side, twist your torso and hips to the left, putting weight on your left foot. Repeat to the right.

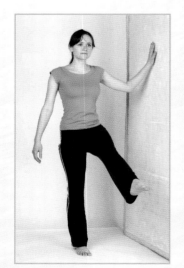
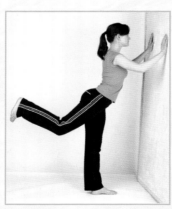

Leg Swings

Do each of these 10–12 times on each leg:

1) Stand sideways with a wall to your left.

2) With weight on your right leg and your left hand on the wall for balance, swing your left leg forward and back.

1) Lean forward with both hands on a wall and your weight on your left leg.

2) Swing your right leg to the left in front of your body, pointing your toes upward as your foot reaches the end of the swing.

3) Swing your right leg back to the right as far as comfortable, again pointing your toes up as your foot reaches the end of the swing.

Warming Up

Many of the same exercises that athletes use as part of their warm-up and cool-down routines are also used for flexibility work. This sometimes leads to confusion between the two. In fact, they are trying to achieve different outcomes (even though they're the same exercises).

Warming Up

When you warm up before hard exercise, you are getting your body ready to perform. Stretching is an important part of any warm-up, but it is doing a different job from in a flexibility session. The aim when warming up is not to increase the joint's range of movement. It is to get the joint working to its full current range of movement.

People used to stretch at the start of their warm-up, but we now know that muscles respond best to stretching exercises after some light activity. This is because the blood is flowing to the muscles more quickly, and the synovial fluid inside the joint has become freer moving. Ten minutes of gentle jogging, swimming, or cycling is a good idea before stretching as part of a warm-up. (Most people then use 10 minutes of dynamic stretches specific to the activity they will be doing, before finishing their warm-up with some work on technique.)

Warming Up for Flexibility Work

Just as for any other training session, athletes warm up before doing flexibility work. They need to get their muscles and joints ready for the session that comes. The warm-up for flexibility work does not need to include

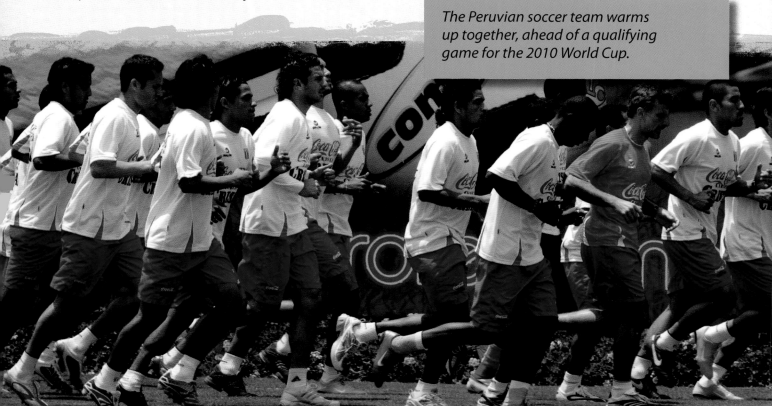

The Peruvian soccer team warms up together, ahead of a qualifying game for the 2010 World Cup.

stretches, however. The stretches come later: they may be the same stretches that are used in a normal warm-up, but this time the aim will be to increase the range of movement in the joint.

Cooling Down

Stretches are an important part of the cool-down sessions athletes do after training. As with a normal warm-up, the aim is not to increase flexibility. It is to help the muscles to recover, and reduce the soreness that may be felt after a hard training session. Static exercises are normally used for cooling down.

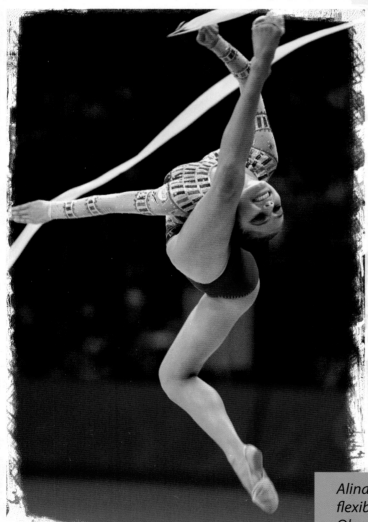

Alina KABAYEVA

Sport: Rhythmic gymnastics
Country: Russia
Born: May 12, 1983

Alina Kabayeva is one of the greatest rhythmic gymnasts the world has ever seen. Famous for her incredible flexibility, she won 25 European Championship medals, 18 World Championship medals, and Olympic gold and silver medals.

When the Russian head coach first saw Kabayeva perform, she said: "I could not believe my eyes… The girl has the rare combination of two qualities crucial in rhythmic gymnastics: flexibility and agility." Kabayeva was soon in the Russian team, and soon winning medals:

- **In 1998, at just 15, Kabayeva won gold at the European Championships. In 1999, she won the title a second time, and followed it with victory at the World Championships.**
- **At the 2004 Olympics, Kabayeva won the gold medal in the all-around competition, and soon afterward retired from gymnastics.**

In 2005, Kabayeva was elected as a member of the State Duma, part of the Russian parliament.

Alina Kabayeva shows jaw-dropping flexibility at the 2000 Sydney Olympic Games.

Hydration and Nutrition

Hydration (what you drink) and nutrition (what you eat) have significant effects on your muscles. These effects are felt mainly in terms of endurance, speed, and strength, but they also affect your flexibility.

Hydration

Not drinking enough has a big effect on sports performance. Once 2 percent of an athlete's body weight has been lost through dehydration, their performance starts to decline. At 4 percent, the ability of the muscles to work decreases. Dehydration ultimately leads to a cramp, in which the muscles tense up and will not immediately relax. At 5 percent of body weight lost, heat exhaustion begins; at 7 percent, the athlete is likely to start hallucinating.

Sports Drinks

Sports drinks help athletes avoid dehydration. These are particularly useful for endurance athletes, whose events may go on for a long time and lead to a lot of fluid being lost as sweat. Most sportspeople find isotonic drinks useful in fighting dehydration. These contain electrolytes (crucial chemicals that are lost in sweat), carbohydrates for energy, and protein to help the muscles repair themselves.

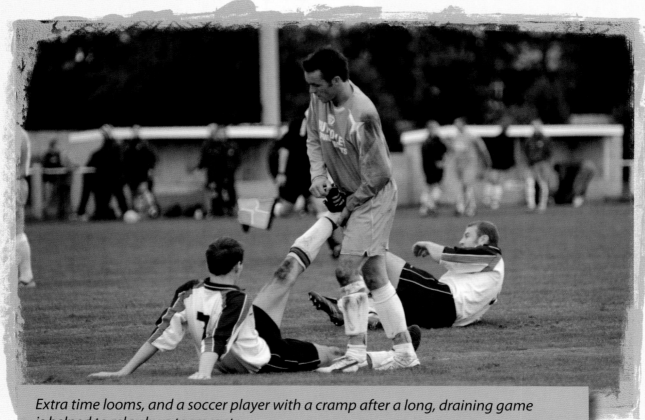

Extra time looms, and a soccer player with a cramp after a long, draining game is helped to relax by a teammate.

Nutrition and Muscle Performance

Nutrition has effects on muscle performance both in the medium and long run. In the medium term, athletes who have not eaten enough will run out of energy to power their muscles. Our muscles store energy in the form of a carbohydrate called glycogen, which the body gets from food. Unless we eat enough carbohydrate-rich food, the muscles do not get enough energy.

In the medium and long run, a second nutrient from food, protein, is also important. Our bodies use protein to build and repair muscle tissue, so eating enough protein-rich food is also crucial to muscles performance.

Rafael Nadal

Sport: Tennis

Country: Spain

Born: June 3, 1986

Rafael Nadal is one of the world's best tennis players. His rivalry with Roger Federer for the World No.1 ranking has lit up tennis tournaments since 2004.

Nadal is famous for his great skill at playing on clay—he is sometimes called the "King of Clay." In 2009, though, he became the first player in history to hold Grand Slam titles on clay, grass, and hard courts at the same time. He took the World No. 1 place from Federer between August 2008 until July 2009—when Federer snatched it back.

Nadal plays an aggressive style of tennis from the baseline of the court, which means he has to run a lot during the match. He is famous for his fitness and speed around the court, as well as his ability to stretch for shots other players might not make.

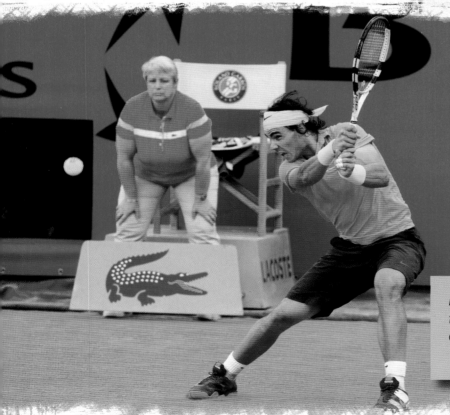

Rafael Nadal powers a shot away from the baseline at the 2009 French Open Championship..

Integrating Flexibility

Flexibility is a crucial part of sports performance, whether for endurance, speed, or power-based events. Because of this, it is not enough to do stretching exercise only as part of your warm-up. At least twice a week, top sportspeople put aside a training session purely to work on their flexibility.

Sport-Specific Flexibility Programs

Most sports have a key set of muscles that play a crucial part in technique. They may provide power, they may be used to get the body into the correct position, or they may do both jobs at once.

Many sports at first seem to use similar muscles: soccer players taking a throw-in and javelin throwers both hurl things through the air, for example. But look in a little more detail, and you see that they use different muscles, in different ways. Like all other sportspeople, they need flexibility programs with three elements:

1) General flexibility, aimed at keeping all joints and muscles able to perform a good range of movement.

2) Sports-type-specific flexibility, for example, exercises aimed at throwers, runners, people who play racket sports, etc.

3) Sport-specific flexibility, which is aimed at the specific movements made by, for example, a sprinter, rugby player, swimmer, or marathon runner.

Sometimes, you don't need a reason to flexible—it's just fun.

Benefits of Improving Flexibility

All athletes gain by working on their flexibility. They will improve their performance, and their technique will become more effective for several key reasons:

- Muscles are more powerful if they are contracted from a relaxed position than from an already-bunched one. So increasing your flexibility will add more power to your technique.

- Inflexible muscles are more likely to pull joints out of alignment, or to be damaged during hard exercise. Increasing flexibility means decreasing the chance of injury.

- Flexible joints and muscles allow ideal joint alignment, making good technique easier to achieve and more efficient.

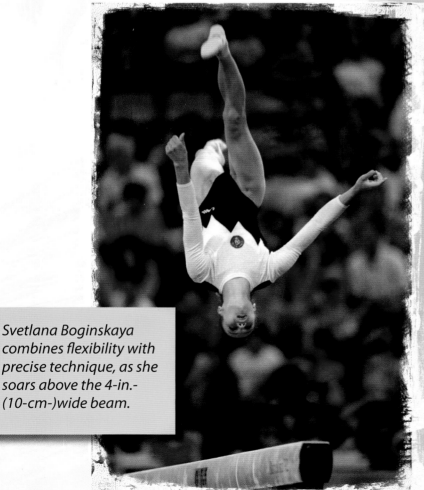

Svetlana Boginskaya combines flexibility with precise technique, as she soars above the 4-in.-(10-cm-)wide beam.

Svetlana Boginskaya

Sport: Artistic gymnastics

Country: Belarus

Born: February 9, 1973

Svetlana Boginskaya is a three-time Olympic champion at artistic gymnastics. Famous for the long-legged grace of her movements, she was sometimes called the "Belorussian Swan."

Boginskaya was a member of her national team by the age of 14. At the 1988 Olympic Games, she won gold medals in the team and vault competitions. It was the start of a long run of success:

- In 1989, she became world champion for the first time. Then, in 1990, Boginskaya became only the third gymnast to win every event at the European Championships.
- At the 1991 World Championships, Boginskaya won gold in the team and balance beam competitions.
- The 1992 Olympics saw her take gold in the team contest.

After the 1992 games Boginskaya retired, then came back to compete for the 1996 Olympics. Only a handful of gymnasts have ever competed at three Olympics Games, but Boginskaya's amazing flexibility meant that she was able to perform techniques even more tricky than in the past. Even so, she did not manage to win a medal.

Testing Your Flexibility

The tests on these pages will give you some idea of how flexible you are. This would be useful in identifying areas to which you need to pay special attention. No athlete, though, can afford to work on just one area of flexibility—even areas that seem good already can still be improved.

Test Tips

These tips will help you get the most from the tests:

- Always warm up in the same way before doing flexibility tests, and do them at the same time of day. This makes comparing results more accurate.

- It is a good idea to test both sides of your body, since there is often a difference between the two.

- Don't forget to breathe out as you relax into each exercise.

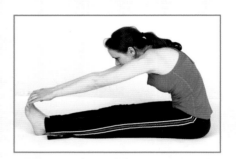

Exercise 2:
Sit on the floor with your legs straight out in front of you. How nearly can you reach your toes?

Poor:	Average:	Good:
More than 6 in. (15 cm) away	4–6 in. (10–15 cm) away	Touching toes

Exercise 3:
Stand up straight. Bend your elbow and reach behind your head and down your spine. With the opposite arm, reach behind your back and up your spine. How near are the fingertips of each hand?

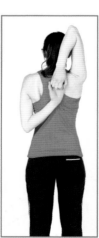

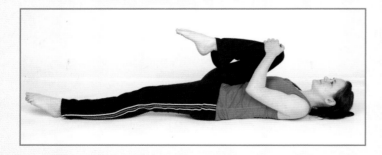

Exercise 1:
Lie on your back on the floor, legs out straight. Lift the knee of one leg toward your chest. How near does it come?

Poor:	Average:	Good:
More than 6 in. (15 cm) from ribs	4–6 in. (10–15 cm) from ribs	Touching ribs

Poor:	Average:	Good:
More than 6 in. (15 cm) apart	4–6 in. (10–15 cm) apart	Touching

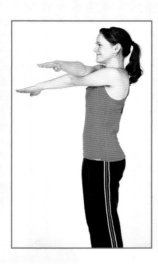

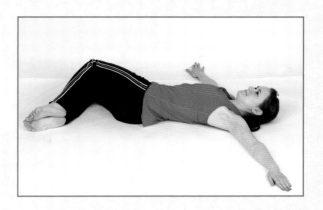

Exercise 4:

Stand up with your arms straight out in front of you, palms facing down. Keeping them straight, try to cross them. At what point do they cross?

Poor:
At the wrist

Average:
At the elbow

Good:
At the upper arm

Exercise 5:

Lie on your back, arms flat on the floor and out to the side, knees bent. Keeping your knees and feet together, twist your torso and lower your knees toward the floor. How close do they get?

Poor:
More than 6 in. (15 cm) away

Average:
4–6 in. (10–15 cm) away

Good:
Resting on the floor

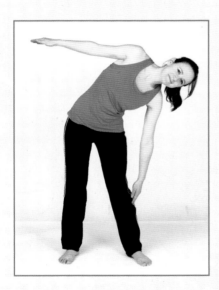

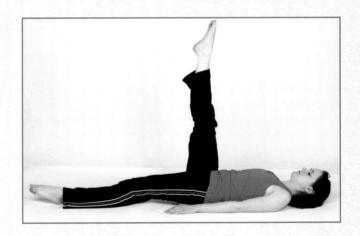

Exercise 6:

Stand with your feet flat and a little more than shoulder-width apart. Reach down the side of your leg (make sure not to lean forward or back). How far do your fingertips go?

Poor:
Above the knee

Average:
Reaching knee

Good:
Below knee

Exercise 7:

Lie on your back, arms by your sides and legs out straight. Lift one leg up straight, from the hip. At what angle does it stop?

Poor:
Less than 90°

Average:
90°

Good:
More than 90°

Glossary

agility
Ability to move quickly and easily from one position to another.

ascent
Climb.

assisted stretching
Stretching done with the help (or assistance) of a partner.

beam
In gymnastics, a beam is a padded strip of wood 4 in. (10 cm) wide, 16.4 ft. (5 m) long, and 4.1 ft. (1.25 m) off the ground.

carbohydrate
Part of food that provides the body with an easily accessed source of energy called glycogen.

central nervous system
Brain and spinal cord, which together control and coordinate the body's movements.

cramp
Involuntary tightening of muscle, often caused by dehydration.

dehydration
Effect of not drinking enough fluids. In humans, dehydration can lead to lessened physical skills, confusion, sickness, and even death.

difficulty rating
Official judgement of how difficult a skill is to perform. In gymnastics, diving, and other sports, the difficulty rating plus the judges' view of how well the skill has been performed produce an athlete's score.

dynamic stretching
Stretching that mimics or replicates the actions performed by muscles and joints during a sport.

electrolytes
Minerals contained in the body, which are crucial for tightening and relaxing muscles.

Grand Slam
In tennis, the Grand Slam tournaments are the Australian Open, the French Open, Wimbledon, and the U.S. Open.

hallucinating
Seeing things that are not actually there.

hard-wired
Programmed in a way that cannot be undone.

isotonic drink
Drinks containing fluid, electrolytes, and 6–8 percent carbohydrates.

joints
Part of the body where bones are connected. Many joints can be moved using muscles; others, such as joints in our skulls, cannot.

mimic
Imitate or copy.

nutrient
Part of food that allows the body to work, and helps it to grow and repair itself.

protein
Nutrient contained in food, which helps the body grow and repair itself.

range of movement
Amount of movement possible from one extreme to the other.

resistance training
A force that slows down something. Resistance training involves asking the muscles to push against extra force, in order to make them stronger.

static stretching
Stretching done alone, by easing into a position and holding it without assistance.

stretch reflex
Safety device that stops muscle from relaxing too far and overextending the joint.

technique
Way of performing an action.

torso
Trunk; central part of body, ending at the neck, shoulders, and hips.

Further Information and Web Sites

BOOKS TO READ

Science Behind Sports: Gymnastics
by Heather Schwartz
(Lucent Books, 2010)

Sports Science
by Andrew Solway
(Heinemann Library, 2009)

Sports Training: The Complete Guide
by John Shepherd
(Firefly Books, 2007)

Yoga Exercises For Teens
by Helen Purperhart
(Hunter House Publishers, 2008)

WEB SITES

Due to the changing nature of Internet links, PowerKids Press has developed an online list of Web sites related to the subject of this book. This site is updated regularly. Please use this link to access this list:
http://www.powerkidslinks.com/tfs/flex

Index